Test

Thyroid Function

Test Your Thyroid Function

Dr. Ray Peat's Guide to Track Your Metabolism and Detect Hypothyroidism

Benedicte Mai Lerche MSc PhD
BiochemNordic

"Healing Metabolism"

Book 2

Copyright © 2023 by Benedicte Mai Lerche, BiochemNordic

All rights reserved, including the right to reproduce this book or portions thereof in any form whatsoever without the prior written permission of the copyright holder. For permissions requests, please e-mail: contact@biochemnordic.com

ISBN: 978-87-975361-4-8 (Hardcover)

ISBN: 978-87-975361-3-1 (Paperback)

ISBN: 978-87-975361-5-5 (E-Book)

A note to the reader:

The author of this book shares research from Dr. Ray Peat and other sources, which may be considered controversial and subject to varying opinions among experts. The content of this book, including but not limited to text, graphics, images, and other material, is offered for informational purposes only and is not intended to replace professional medical advice, diagnosis, or treatment. Readers are strongly encouraged to consult with their physician or another qualified health provider for any questions related to a medical condition or health concerns. Neither the author nor the publisher makes any express or implied representations or warranties concerning the information's suitability, reliability, timeliness, or accuracy. The author and publisher are not responsible for any consequences resulting from the use or misuse of the information in this book. They specifically disclaim any liability for personal or other loss, risk, or harm that may be incurred, directly or indirectly, as a result of using or applying any content of this book. Readers should be aware that applying this information to their lives is a personal decision and responsibility.

Book Series

Through my "Healing Metabolism" book series, I am dedicated to sharing Dr. Ray Peat's health research. The series aims to deepen readers' understanding and offer practical methods for overcoming metabolic and hormonal imbalances, utilizing diet, thyroid replacement therapy, hormonal support compounds, and other lifestyle changes.

Book 1:
The first book, "How I Overcame Hypothyroidism," chronicles my personal health journey and victory over low thyroid function (hypothyroidism) using Dr. Ray Peat's health approach. It introduces Dr. Peat's research and equips readers with a fundamental understanding of his key health concepts for healing metabolism.

Book 2:
The current book "Test Your Thyroid Function" is designed to help you understand Dr. Ray Peat's principles for tracking your metabolism and detecting hypothyroidism. You'll learn how to accurately interpret your thyroid lab test results and how to use pulse rate and body temperature to monitor your metabolism at home. This book also

covers essential aspects of thyroid function and metabolic health.

Book 3:
In the third book, "How to Boost Metabolism with Food," you will learn how to apply Dr. Ray Peat's dietary principles to enhance your metabolic rate. Many people unknowingly consume foods that slow down their metabolism. This book helps you identify these foods while introducing delicious alternatives that promote thyroid health and a faster metabolism.

Future volumes:
I am developing further volumes for the "Healing Metabolism" series. Upcoming books will provide insights into topics such as thyroid medication and hormonal support supplements like progesterone and pregnenolone.

Support my work:
If you find any of my books helpful, I would be extremely grateful if you could take a few minutes to leave a short review on the platform where you purchased the book or on Goodreads. This will help other potential readers dealing with similar health issues discover and benefit from my work.

Contents

Dedication 1

Introduction 3

Chapter 1: Thyroid Physiology 7

    The Thyroid Gland 9

    Interplay of T4, T3, and TSH 11

    The Importance of T3 13

Chapter 2: Hypothyroidism 15

    Hypothyroid Symptoms 17

    Causes of Hypothyroidism 23

    Understanding reverse T3 29

    Hashimoto's Thyroiditis 33

    Triggers of Hypothyroidism 35

Chapter 3: Thyroid Labs 37

    Thyroid Blood Tests 39

    Historical Aspects 41

    What is a Good TSH Level? 43

    Free or Total T4 and T3 47

    Dr. Peat's Thyroid Blood Tests 51

    Ratio of T3 to rT3 53

    Thyroid Antibody Levels...................................55

    Biotin and Blood Test 59

    Thyroid Meds and Blood Tests.......................61

    Thyroid Blood Test Summary.........................65

    Thyroid Blood Tests Table 69

Chapter 4: At-Home Thyroid Testing.................73

    Comprehensive Testing....................................75

    Body Temperature 77

    Pulse Rate 85

    Effect of Stress Hormones................................89

    Measuring Temperature...................................95

    Measuring Pulse Rate 97

    A Note on Wearables 99

    Pulse and Temp Summary.............................101

    Pulse and Temp Table 105

Chapter 5: Track your Thyroid Function 107

    Pulse, Temp, Symptoms Logs 109

Chapter 6: Healing Metabolism..........................119

    Dr. Ray Peat's Health Method......................121

Your Review Matters	125
About the Author	127
References	129

Benedicte Mai Lerche MSc PhD

Dedication

With deep appreciation, this book is dedicated to the memory of the late Dr. Ray Peat, whose exceptional research and invaluable guidance were instrumental in my recovery from hypothyroidism and the restoration of my health.

Raymond Franklin Peat (1936-2022), a distinguished American scholar with a Ph.D. in biology, dedicated over half a century to investigating the intricate relationship between nutrition, hormones, and health. His pioneering contributions in the fields of metabolism and thyroid function have left an indelible impact on countless lives, including my own.

Dr. Ray Peat viewed optimal thyroid function as a fundamental element of overall wellness. He contended that many individuals were experiencing a variety of symptoms that could be effectively addressed through accurate diagnosis and targeted treatment of hypothyroidism.

In his extensive research, Dr. Peat examined topics such as the best dietary practices for promoting thyroid health, effective thyroid medications, and the role of related hormones like natural progesterone and pregnenolone.

The goal of this book is to provide a thorough yet accessible explanation of Dr. Ray Peat's diagnostic techniques for hypothyroidism. It explores his perspectives on interpreting thyroid blood tests and elaborates on his method of using pulse and temperature metrics in conjunction with symptom analysis for a comprehensive assessment of thyroid functionality.

Benedicte Mai Lerche
December 2023

Introduction

In my early twenties, I faced the significant challenge of severe hypothyroidism, also known as underactive thyroid function or low metabolism. Confronted with debilitating symptoms and in pursuit of effective treatment, I embarked on a transformative journey that reshaped my life.

I was fortunate to encounter Dr. Ray Peat, a renowned expert in nutrition, metabolism, and hormonal health. Discovering his work marked a turning point in my battle with hypothyroidism, providing the crucial knowledge I needed to regain my health.

Following Dr. Peat's advice, I adopted dietary changes, thyroid medications, and hormonal supplements, which all helped revitalize my metabolism.

Inspired by my recovery, I pursued biochemistry in university and later founded my website, biochemnordic.com. Here, and in my book series "Healing Metabolism", I share Dr. Peat's health principles and offer insights into nutrition, metabolism, and hormones.

For more on my health journey and how I applied Dr. Peat's philosophies, I invite you to read my first book, "How I Overcame Hypothyroidism".

This second book aims to deepen your understanding of Dr. Peat's views on thyroid testing and his methods for detecting Hypothyroidism.

The book is structured as follows:

Chapter 1: Lays the foundation for understanding thyroid physiology, detailing the role of the thyroid gland and the interplay between thyroid hormones (T4, T3) and TSH, with a focus on the active thyroid hormone, T3.

Chapter 2: Delves into the consequences of underactive thyroid function, reflecting Dr. Ray Peat's insights on various causes of hypothyroidism and their effects on the body. It offers a detailed list of symptoms associated with hypothyroidism and discusses the common triggers for this condition. Additionally, the chapter addresses the role of reverse T3 (rT3) and explores Hashimoto's thyroiditis.

Chapter 3: Delves into thyroid blood tests, providing historical context for the reference ranges of thyroid function tests. It explains the crucial distinction between 'reference ranges' and 'optimal ranges' for these tests, emphasizing that hypothyroidism can still be present even if blood test results are within the 'normal' range. The chapter includes recommendations for reliable thyroid blood tests, aimed at enhancing communication with your healthcare provider. Additionally, it offers guidance on interpreting test results, helping readers gain a deeper understanding of their thyroid function.

Chapter 4: Discusses methods for assessing thyroid function at the cellular level, using pulse rate and body temperature as key indicators. The effect of stress hormones on these measurements is clarified. Detailed guidelines for tracking pulse and temperature are provided. The chapter also discusses different types of devices suitable for these measurements.

Chapter 5: Introduces schemas specifically designed to aid in tracking your pulse and temperature daily, as well as over time, along with a dedicated checklist for assessing symptoms related to hypothyroidism. These tools are invaluable for methodically monitoring and comprehending the changes in your thyroid function.

Chapter 6: Provides an introductory overview of Dr. Ray Peat's health philosophy, along with basic guidance for addressing hypothyroidism. It briefly outlines his fundamental ideas, effectively setting the stage for further exploration. This chapter serves as a stepping stone for those interested in delving deeper into Dr. Peat's methodologies in future readings or research

Benedicte Mai Lerche MSc PhD

Chapter 1: Thyroid Physiology

Benedicte Mai Lerche MSc PhD

The Thyroid Gland

To delve into the realm of thyroid testing, it's essential to first grasp key facets of thyroid physiology. This chapter is dedicated precisely to that purpose.

Thyroid function refers to metabolism or the metabolic rate, which is a medical term indicating the process through which cells convert food into energy (Barnes & Galton, 1976, p. 3).

Metabolism is regulated by the thyroid hormones, which are produced and released by the thyroid gland (Society of Endocrinology, 2020).

Located in the front of the throat, the human thyroid gland (Figure 1) has a butterfly shape (Barnes & Galton, 1976, p. 3). It is a small endocrine gland that produces and releases triiodothyronine (T3), the active thyroid hormone, and thyroxine (T4), a prohormone or storage hormone.

Collectively, T4 and T3 are known as the thyroid hormones (Society of Endocrinology, 2020). The thyroid gland is known to secrete more T4 than T3 (American Thyroid Association, 2023a). As per Dr. Ray Peat, T4 and T3 are released in a ratio of about

3:1, which corresponds to 75% T4 and 25% T3 (Peat, 2001a, p. 73).

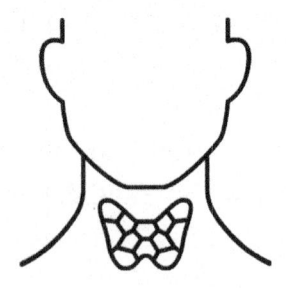

Figure 1: A sketch of the human thyroid gland, illustrating its distinctive butterfly shape and its location at the front of the throat.

Interplay of T4, T3, and TSH

Thyroid-stimulating hormone (TSH), originating from the pituitary gland in the brain, stimulates the thyroid gland to produce and release thyroid hormones into the bloodstream (Society of Endocrinology, 2020); (Vander, et al., 2001, p. 280).

The thyroid hormones and TSH operate within a negative feedback loop, which is illustrated in Figure 2, see below.

A low TSH level serves as an indicator of adequate blood levels of T4 and T3. Conversely, when T4 and T3 levels decrease, it triggers an increase in TSH (Vander, et al., 2001, p. 281).

Consequently, the TSH value is utilized as a means to evaluate the function of the thyroid gland (Peat, 2008, p. 2). I will return to the issue of measuring blood levels of TSH, T4, and T3 later in this book.

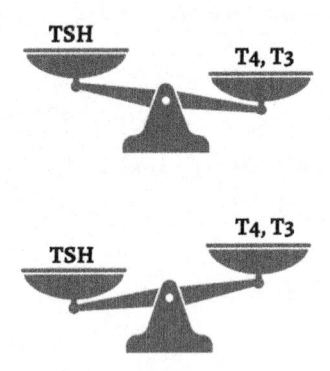

Figure 2: Demonstrating the relationship between TSH and thyroid hormones (T4 and T3). Inadequate levels of T4 and T3 result in an increase in TSH levels, as shown in the first image. While optimal levels of these hormones cause a decrease in TSH, as depicted in the second image.

The Importance of T3

When discussing metabolism, it is crucial to always keep in mind that T3 is the active thyroid hormone, which affects cells and regulates metabolism, whereas T4 is a pro-hormone for T3 (Society of Endocrinology, 2020).

Once secreted by the thyroid gland, T4 can be converted to the active thyroid hormone T3 by specific enzymes in other organs and tissues (Society of Endocrinology, 2020). Most of this conversion occurs in the liver, which allows the liver to regulate thyroid function (Peat, 2001a, p. 73).

T3's main function is to energize cells, thereby facilitating the essential life processes of the body's tissues and organs (Vander, et al., 2001, p. 267).

T3 controls the metabolic rate, which refers to the speed at which cells utilize oxygen ($6O_2$) to transform nutrients into carbon dioxide (CO_2), water (H_2O), heat, and adenosine triphosphate (ATP), the latter serves as a biological form of energy.

To exemplify, consider the metabolic process involving glucose, represented by the following equation (Vander, et al., 2001, pp. 619-620; Boston University School of Public Health, 2017):

$$C_6H_{12}O_6 + 6O_2 \rightarrow 6CO_2 + 6H_2O + Heat + ATP$$

ATP acts as an energy source within the body, powering essential cellular functions and reactions (Vander, et al., 2001, pp. 619-620).

Peat highlighted the critical importance of abounded energy for maintaining the correct structure and functionality of the body's tissues and organs (Peat, 2001a, pp. 1-5).

He proposed that diseases arise when there's an imbalance between the body's energy supply and the demands of its environment (Peat, 2001a, pp. 1-5). Specifically, he pointed out that hypothyroidism, marked by low energy levels, is instrumental in triggering harmful degenerative processes (Peat, 2001d, p. 16). Since hypothyroidism impacts all cells and tissues, it presents a range of symptoms. The next chapter provides a detailed list of symptoms associated with reduced thyroid function.

Chapter 2: Hypothyroidism

Benedicte Mai Lerche MSc PhD

Hypothyroid Symptoms

The severe forms of hypothyroidism, known as cretinism in infants and children, and myxedema in adults, have a profound impact on the body. They affect all tissues and organs, leading to devastating health outcomes (Barnes & Galton, 1976, pp. 20-22). However, it's important to note that severe hypothyroidism is relatively uncommon (Barnes & Galton, 1976, pp. 20-22).

In contrast, milder forms of hypothyroidism are more common and can present with subtle symptoms. They may affect various body systems, though not necessarily to the same extent in each individual. As a result, manifestations of an underactive thyroid can vary from person to person (Barnes & Galton, 1976, pp. 22-25)

In fact, it's not uncommon for individuals to have hypothyroidism without being aware of it. This lack of awareness may lead to attempts to manage individual symptoms without identifying the underlying cause.

Below is a list of common symptoms associated with hypothyroidism (Barnes & Galton, 1976, pp. 22-24;

Wilson, 2015, p. 25; Peat, 2001d, pp. 16-18; Peat, 2001b, p. 78).

This list, while not exhaustive, provides an overview of the diverse symptoms related to low thyroid function. It's important to remember that not all symptoms need to be present for a diagnosis of hypothyroidism.

Common hypothyroidism symptoms:

Fatigue: Feeling tired and lacking energy, even after getting adequate rest (chronic fatigue).

Headaches: Experiencing pressure headaches and migraines.

Hypoglycemia: Having low blood sugar, resulting in a need to eat frequently to avoid feeling faint and dizzy.

Weight changes: Experiencing unexplained weight gain or difficulty losing weight despite maintaining a healthy diet and regular exercise routine. Some individuals may also experience weight loss.

Low body temperature: Having cold intolerance, feeling excessively cold even in warm temperatures, and having cold hands and feet.

Reduced heart rate: Experiencing a slow heart rate (bradycardia) and decreased heart function.

Heart problems & disease: Experiencing heart pain, poor heart sounds, enlargement of the heart, palpitations, and hypertension.

Constipation: Experiencing slow digestion, difficulty passing stools, and infrequent bowel movements.

Digestive problems: Painful digestion, irritable bowel syndrome (IBS), as well as an overgrowth of bad bacteria and candida.

Dry skin: Having dry, rough, thin, pale skin that may be itchy and scaly, accompanied by conditions like eczema or skin infections.

Brittle hair & nails: Experiencing thinning of hair and nails, hair loss, changes in hair texture, and potential loss of the outer third of the eyebrows.

Muscle and joint pain: Experiencing muscle aches, stiffness, and joint pain not attributed to any specific injury or physical activity.

Carpal tunnel syndrome: Having pain, numbness, and tingling sensations in the hand, arms, and fingers (carpal tunnel syndrome).

Mood changes: Experiencing depression, anxiety, irritability, and mood swings.

Cognitive impairment: Having difficulty concentrating, poor memory, and decreased mental alertness (brain fog).

Hoarseness: Experiencing a deepening or hoarse voice, often accompanied by a sore throat.

Swelling: Experiencing water retention (edema), often with swelling or puffiness in the face, hands, feet, or ankles.

High cholesterol: Having elevated levels of cholesterol in the blood, even with a healthy diet and lifestyle.

Decreased libido: Experiencing a loss of interest in sexual activity and a reduced sexual drive.

Menstrual irregularities: Having irregular menstrual cycles, heavy menstrual bleeding, prolonged menstrual periods, painful menstruation, and experiencing symptoms of premenstrual syndrome (PMS) and polycystic ovaries (PCOS).

Infertility & miscarriage: Experiencing male and female infertility, with a higher chance of miscarriage in females.

Insomnia: Having problems falling asleep and/or waking up during the night.

Other symptoms: Poor vision, hearing loss, anemia, allergies, frequent colds, infections, orange calluses, inflammation, premature aging, and more.

Benedicte Mai Lerche MSc PhD

Causes of Hypothyroidism

Dr. Ray Peat identified several factors that can lead to hypothyroidism. Three common causes include inadequate secretion of thyroid hormones by the thyroid gland (Sluggish Gland), ineffective conversion of T4 to active thyroid hormone T3 (Conversion Defect), or impaired cellular response to T3 (T3 Blockage) (Peat, 2001a, pp. 72-74; Wilson, 2015, pp. 24-28).

A Sluggish Thyroid Gland:

An underactive thyroid gland is unable to produce sufficient amounts of the thyroid hormones T4 and T3. This deficiency might be attributed to the gland's intrinsic limitations. However, other factors like diet and estrogen dominance can also play a role in diminishing its hormonal output (Peat, 2001b, pp. 155-156).

Dr. Ray Peat highlighted, that polyunsaturated fats, which are prevalent in various liquid cooking oils, impair thyroid function in several ways. These fats disrupt the thyroid gland's ability to synthesize and release hormones (Peat, 2001b, pp. 155-156).

Vegetables from the cabbage family, also known as Brassicaceae or Cruciferae — which include cabbage, broccoli, cauliflower, Brussels sprouts, and kale — contain compounds called goitrogens (Peat, 2001b, p. 78; Everyday Health, 2018).

Goitrogens can adversely affect thyroid health by hindering the thyroid gland's ability to absorb iodine, an essential element for the synthesis of thyroid hormones (Cleveland Clinic, 2019).

Furthermore, estrogen can impede the release of hormones from the thyroid gland (Peat, 2001b, p. 78). During significant life stages like puberty, pregnancy, and menopause the thyroid gland often enlarges, possibly due to estrogen dominance, which can lead to the entrapment of thyroid hormones within the gland (Peat, 2001a, p. 74).

Conversion Defect:

Sometimes, people have high levels of T4 yet still experience symptoms of hypothyroidism. This situation likely occurs due to inefficient conversion of T4 to T3 (Peat, 2001a, p. 74).

As previously noted, the liver is the primary organ responsible for converting T4 to T3. Consequently, compromised liver function can lead to hypothyroidism (Peat, 2001a, p. 73).

Typically, women have less robust liver function compared to men, in part due to the adverse effects of estrogen on liver activity. Consequently, this makes the conversion of T4 to T3 more challenging for women (Peat, 2001a, p. 74).

Factors like a diet deficient in good quality protein and B-vitamins can also impair liver function, and thereby limit the production of T3 (Ray Peat Clips, 2016e).

Low blood sugar (hypoglycemia) and a lack of selenium are also known to impede the conversion of T4 to T3 (Peat, 2001a, pp. 73-75; Wilson, 2015, p. 26).

The production of T3 is further compromised by physical or mental stress, as stress hormones (cortisol and adrenaline) directly interfere with the T4 to T3 conversion process (Peat, 2008, p. 3).

T3 Blockage:

Dr. Ray Peat emphasized that even if an individual has sufficient levels of T3, they may still experience symptoms of hypothyroidism. This can be attributed to decreased tissue sensitivity to T3, for example, from a diet high in polyunsaturated fats (Peat, 2001a, p. 72).

Polyunsaturated fats not only disrupt the synthesis and release of T4 and T3 by the thyroid gland, but they also impair the transport of these hormones in the bloodstream and block the action of T3 at the cellular level (Peat, 2001b, p. 156).

Stress affects not only the conversion of T4 to T3, but high levels of stress hormones can also lead to increased production of reverse T3 (rT3), which can block the function of T3, thereby undermining thyroid function at the cellular level (Peat, 2008, p. 3).

Table 1 below shows the three common causes of hypothyroidism and how they affect blood levels of T4, T3, and TSH individually.

Causes of Hypothyroidism	T3	T4	TSH
Sluggish Gland	Low	Low	High
Conversion Defect	Low	High	Normal
T3 Blockage	Normal	Normal	Normal

Table 1: Three common causes of hypothyroidism according to Dr. Ray Peat.

Dr. Peat's comprehensive research suggests that hypothyroidism is frequently a result of a combination of the three factors outlined in Table 1.

Regardless of the specific underlying cause, hypothyroidism ultimately leads to an energy deficiency within the body, manifesting as hypothyroid symptoms (Peat, 2001a, pp. 72-74; Peat, 2008, pp. 2-3).

Before delving into thyroid blood testing, subsequent sections will cover the role of reverse T3 (rT3). I will also examine Dr. Ray Peat's views on Hashimoto's thyroiditis and explore common triggers of hypothyroidism.

Understanding reverse T3

Reverse T3, also known as rT3, is an inactive form of T3 that acts as a metabolic suppressor by chemically inhibiting the activity of the active thyroid hormone T3 (Peat, 2001d, p. 20; Peat, 2008, p. 3).

As illustrated in Figure 3, T4 is normally converted into the active thyroid hormone T3. In typical circumstances, a negligible amount of T4 is also changed into rT3, but this conversion is minimal in healthy people (Alan Jacobs, 2023).

```
        ┌─────────────────┐
        │       T4        │
        │ Storage Hormone │
        └─────────────────┘
           ↙           ↘
┌─────────────────┐  ┌─────────────────┐
│       T3        │  │   Reverse T3    │
│  Active Hormone │  │    Blocks T3    │
└─────────────────┘  └─────────────────┘
```

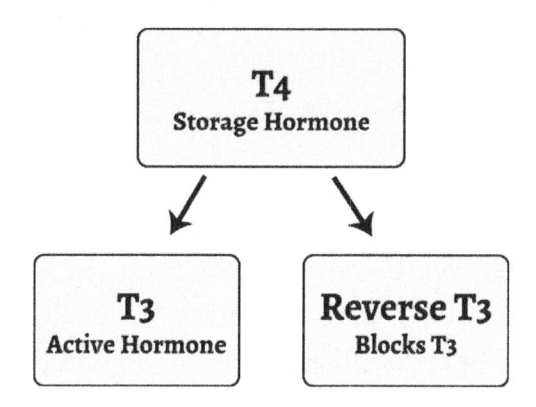

Figure 3: Illustrates the conversion of T4 into T3 and reverse T3 (rT3), where rT3 blocks T3's action, yet its production remains minimal in healthy individuals.

When produced in excess, rT3 becomes problematic as it binds to T3 receptors but unlike T3 fails to stimulate metabolic activity (Mary Shomon, 2023a; Health Central, 2021).

In essence, the role of reverse rT3 is to bind to thyroid receptors without activating them. This action prevents T3 from binding to these receptors, ultimately disrupting the usual metabolic processes normally facilitated by T3 (Mary Shomon, 2023a; Health Central, 2021).

The body is known to ramp up the production of rT3 during crisis situations such as critical illness, extreme dieting, or starvation (Mary Shomon, 2022; Alan Jacobs, 2023).

Stress, and specifically the stress hormones adrenaline and cortisol, can increase the production of rT3 (Peat, 2008, p. 3; Ray Peat Clips, 2016a).

While the full significance of rT3 is not yet clearly understood, it is thought to serve as a mechanism to slow metabolism and preserve the body's energy stores in times of stress or scarcity (Mary Shomon, 2023b; Mary Shomon, 2022).

In the next chapter, I will delve into the importance of measuring rT3 levels in the blood and how to compare these levels with T3 to determine the true amount of active T3 available in the body.

Benedicte Mai Lerche MSc PhD

Hashimoto's Thyroiditis

First identified by Dr. Haruko Hashimoto in 1912, Hashimoto's thyroiditis, also known as chronic lymphocytic thyroiditis or autoimmune thyroiditis, represents an autoimmune variation of hypothyroidism (Harvard medical School, 2019).

This autoimmune form of hypothyroidism is most commonly found in women and is marked by a thyroid gland that becomes populated with white blood cells (Ray Peat KMUD, 2013; Harvard medical School, 2019).

In autoimmune disorders like Hashimoto's thyroiditis, the immune system targets its own tissues, in this instance, the thyroid gland. Symptoms frequently include an enlarged thyroid gland, or goiter, which is unable to produce enough hormones (Harvard medical School, 2019; Ray Peat KMUD, 2013)

Blood tests usually reveal low levels of T4 and T3, elevated TSH, and the existence of thyroid antibodies, such as thyroid peroxidase antibodies (TPOAb, Anti-TPO) and thyroglobulin antibodies (TgAb) (HealthCentral, 2014). Most people with Hashimoto's will have an elevation of one or both of these antibodies (Wentz, 2023b).

The general medical understanding is that these thyroid antibodies can impair the function of the thyroid gland, inhibiting the production of thyroid hormones, which eventually can cause hypothyroidism (Very Well Health, 2023a).

Contradicting conventional medical perspectives, Dr. Peat posited that thyroid antibodies should not be considered the cause of this form of hypothyroidism. Rather, he interpreted their presence as a sign that the body's repair mechanisms are trying to heal the thyroid gland (Ray Peat KMUD, 2013).

Dr. Peat generally classifies Hashimoto's thyroiditis as a subset of hypothyroidism, with similar symptoms and treatment requirements (Ray Peat KMUD, 2013).

The upcoming chapter will focus on thyroid blood testing, covering various aspects including thyroid antibody levels. However, before we dive into this, the next section will explore the triggers of hypothyroidism.

Triggers of Hypothyroidism

Based on my work with clients, I've observed that factors frequently cited as contributing to the onset of hypothyroidism include poor dietary choices and various kinds of stress—either mental or physical.

Common triggers include fasting, sustained protein deficiency, and eating foods known to negatively affect the thyroid.

Stress factors such as excessive aerobic workouts, work-related stress, difficult relationships, or severe bacterial and viral infections are often observed among those who develop hypothyroidism.

Numerous health-conscious individuals might inadvertently adopt lifestyle choices that impede metabolism. This could include engaging in excessive strenuous exercises and consuming foods like beans, lentils, nuts, polyunsaturated fats, and undercooked cruciferous vegetables such as broccoli, cauliflower, and cabbage—all known to negatively affect thyroid function (Peat, 2001a, p. 75)

While some individuals may have mildly low thyroid levels in their medical history, significant issues often do not surface until they engage in a poor diet or encounter specific stressors.

Dr. Ray Peat recommended not getting too absorbed in treating the specific triggers that lead to hypothyroidism. Many individuals, including myself, often devote excessive attention to fighting off viral and bacterial infections. I've observed numerous people spending years on various treatment protocols aimed at eradicating a specific virus or bacteria, believing that these infections are the root cause of their health issues.

However, Dr. Peat advocated for a shift in focus, advising people to move away from endlessly treating these individual triggers. Instead, he encourages removing oneself from harmful environments and focusing on diet and lifestyle practices that improve thyroid function and hormonal balance. By adopting this approach, individuals can optimize their body's healing capabilities.

Benedicte Mai Lerche MSc PhD

Chapter 3: Thyroid Labs

Benedicte Mai Lerche MSc PhD

Thyroid Blood Tests

Blood tests are essential for evaluating thyroid function, but it's crucial to consider multiple factors before relying solely on their results. In this section, I will provide an overview of various aspects of thyroid blood testing, with further elaboration in the subsequent sections of this chapter.

In assessing thyroid function, medical professionals may perform blood tests for TSH, T4, T3, reverse T3 (rT3), and thyroid antibodies (Peat, 2008, p. 2; Peat, 2000, pp. 1-4; Peat, 2001a, p. 74).

Doctors often opt to measure the unbound, or free, forms of T4 and T3, rather than the total amounts of these hormones. However, Dr. Ray Peat has argued that this method of measuring free thyroid hormones lacks biological justification (Peat, 2000, pp. 3-4).

Although the reverse T3 (rT3) blood test is available and regarded as significant by some physicians, including Dr. Ray Peat (Ray Peat Clips, 2021), it is infrequently carried out in practice (Mary Shomon, 2022; Mary Shomon, 2023b; Mary Shomon, 2023a)

It is also important to recognize that the reference ranges for thyroid blood tests are quite broad. This implies that an individual must be severely hypothyroid before their levels fall outside these so-called 'normal' ranges (Peat, 2008, p. 2; Peat, 2000, pp. 1-2).

This chapter delves into the differentiation between optimal and normal test ranges, thereby aiding in the accurate interpretation of lab results.

It is also important to emphasize that blood tests may not accurately reflect cellular thyroid activity, as they only measure the levels of hormones in the bloodstream, not their impact on cells (Peat, 2001a, p. 72; Wilson, 2015, p. 28).

In the remainder of this chapter, I will delve deeper into these key aspects of thyroid blood testing. The aim is to enhance your understanding of your own test results and facilitate meaningful discussions with your healthcare provider. Additionally, you have the opportunity to discuss your test results in a counseling session with me

Historical Aspects

Before World War II, the diagnosis of hypothyroidism involved an extensive list of signs and symptoms, along with the measurement of basal metabolic rate (BMR) (Peat, 2000, p. 1; Peat, 2008, p. 1).

As mentioned in Chapter 1, T3 regulates the metabolic rate, which is the rate at which cells use oxygen to convert nutrients into energy (Vander, et al., 2001, pp. 619-620).

The BMR test assesses this process by measuring an individual's oxygen consumption rate at rest. It provides an estimate of the calories burned to maintain basic life processes, essentially offering a measure of thyroid function (Garnet Health, 2016; Pediatric On Call, 2023; Cleveland Clinic, 2023).

In the late 1940s, a new diagnostic method for hypothyroidism, the protein-bound iodine (PBI) test, was introduced (Peat, 2000, p. 1). This test led to a significant decrease in diagnosed hypothyroid cases, indicating that only 5% of the population had the condition (Peat, 2000, p. 1).
By the 1960s, the limitations of the PBI test became apparent, and it was no longer considered a reliable

metric for measuring thyroid function. Nevertheless, the notion that only 5% of the population was affected by hypothyroidism had already taken root (Peat, 2000, p. 2).

When the TSH blood test was first introduced, the prevailing notion that only 5% of the population had hypothyroidism influenced the standard reference ranges for this new test, leading to the acceptance of dangerously high TSH levels as normal (Peat, 2000, pp. 1-2).

Many individuals who display symptoms of hypothyroidism test within the standard reference range for TSH, thereby evading a diagnosis of hypothyroidism (Peat, 2000, pp. 1-2; Peat, 2008, p. 2). In the following section, I will explore TSH as an indicator of thyroid function in greater detail.

What is a Good TSH Level?

As discussed in Chapter 1, thyroid hormones and TSH operate within a negative feedback loop.

A low TSH level indicates adequate blood levels of T4 and T3. Conversely, when T4 and T3 levels decline, there is an increase in TSH secretion. Therefore, TSH blood level is used as a metric to assess the functionality of the thyroid gland (Vander, et al., 2001, p. 281; Peat, 2008, p. 2).

One might reasonably assume that the body could use this feedback loop to correct hypothyroidism by elevating TSH levels. This, in turn, would prompt the thyroid gland to function more vigorously and produce more thyroid hormone (Vander, et al., 2001, p. 281).

However, it is crucial to understand that TSH itself possesses pro-inflammatory qualities (Ray Peat Clips, 2016c), and overstimulation by TSH can lead to disorganization within the thyroid gland (Peat, 2000, p. 2). Dr. Ray Peat emphasized that many symptoms associated with hypothyroidism actually stem directly from the elevated TSH itself (Ray Peat, Clips, 2016b; Peat, 2008, p. 2; Ray Peat Clips, 2016c).

The crucial issue is determining the TSH threshold that indicates an underactive thyroid gland (Peat, 2008, p. 2). However, there is disagreement among experts regarding the upper limit for TSH (Faix, 2013).

TSH is measured in milli International Units per Liter (mIU/L)

According to the American Association of Clinical Endocrinologists, the upper limit for TSH is set at 3 mIU/L (Peat, 2008, p. 2). Some specialists suggest a limit no higher than 2.5 mIU/L (Faix, 2013), while Dr. Ray Peat advocated for a TSH level below 1 mIU/L (Peat, 2008, p. 2).

However, in many countries, the accepted upper threshold for TSH is set at 4, and sometimes even 5 mIU/L (Health, UCLA, 2023).

Dr. Ray Peat emphasized that he never encountered a person with a TSH level over 2 mIU/L who was in good health. This observation led him to conclude that a normal or healthy TSH level should be below 1 (Peat, 2008, p. 2). This view is echoed by some integrative health experts, who suggest that optimal well-being is often associated with a TSH level at or below 1 mIU/mL (Wentz, 2023b).

Additionally, Dr. Peat noted that effective management of some types of thyroid cancer may involve fully suppressing TSH levels (Peat, 2008, p. 2). He cited research indicating that maintaining TSH levels below 0.4 mIU/L could offer protection against thyroid cancer, suggesting that a safe TSH range might be as low as 0 to 0.4 mIU/L (Ray Peat, Clips, 2016b).

Dr. Peat had no reservations about maintaining notably low TSH levels. He argued that such levels could act as a protective mechanism against various health issues, given the pro-inflammatory nature of TSH itself (Peat, 2008, p. 2).

Moreover, Dr. Peat stressed that there is no scientific evidence indicating negative consequences from maintaining low TSH levels. He concluded that there is no justification for establishing a lower limit for the TSH reference range (Peat, 2008, p. 2; Ray Peat Clips, 2016c).

When evaluating TSH levels, it's crucial to acknowledge that factors other than thyroid hormones can affect TSH suppression. For example, sustained high levels of cortisol, the stress hormone, can inhibit TSH secretion (Peat, 2008, p. 3).

This introduces complexity in using TSH as an indicator of thyroid function. Many individuals with hypothyroidism may increase the production of stress hormones to compensate for their lack of energy (Peat, 2008, p. 5).

As a result, TSH levels might appear normal or even low, despite the presence of hypothyroidism. Thus, relying on TSH as the sole metric for thyroid function assessment can be misleading (Peat, 2008, p. 3).

In the following sections of this chapter, I will explore additional blood tests that are instrumental in evaluating thyroid function.

Free or Total T4 and T3

As described in Chapter 1, the human thyroid gland releases approximately 75% thyroxine (T4) and 25% triiodothyronine (T3) (Peat, 2001a, p. 73).

T3 is the active thyroid hormone, while T4 is a prohormone for T3 (Society of Endocrinology, 2020).

The majority of T4 and T3 hormones circulate in the blood bound to proteins, with only a small fraction existing as free hormones (Health, UCLA, 2023).

When conducting blood tests for T3 and T4, medical professionals can evaluate either the total or the free forms of these hormones (Health, UCLA, 2023; American Thyroid Association, 2023a):

- o Total T4 measures both bound and free T4.
- o Free T4 measures only unbound T4.
- o Total T3 measures both bound and free T3.
- o Free T3 measures only unbound T3.

On test results, these are typically labeled as T4, free T4 (or FT4), T3, and free T3 (or FT3).

The term 'total' is usually omitted. However, if 'free' or 'F' is indicated, it signifies the measurement of the unbound form of the hormone.

The free hormone hypothesis suggests that only the non-bound fraction of a hormone can exert biological effects (Bikle, 2021). Consequently, some medical professionals believe that measuring free T4 and free T3 is the most effective way to assess thyroid function (Grant, 2019).

However, Dr. Ray Peat contended that the free hormone hypothesis erroneously assumes that hormones become biologically inactive when bound to proteins. He further clarified that, in the case of thyroid hormones, the protein-bound forms are, in fact, biologically active (Peat, 2000, pp. 3-4).

Dr. Peat expressed concerns regarding the measurement of free T4 and free T3, noting that these levels might not accurately reflect the true biological activity of thyroid hormones in the body. Such a mismatch between measurement results and actual biological effects could present challenges in correlating thyroid-related symptoms with blood test results (Peat, 2000, p. 3).

According to Dr. Ray Peat, measuring free thyroid hormones is primarily a laboratory construct, and its significance in interpreting thyroid function should be minimized (Peat, 2008, p. 6).

Dr. Peat advocated for measuring total T4 and T3 instead of their free forms.

Furthermore, it's important to note that some medical professionals refrain from performing the free T3 blood test, viewing it as too unreliable and thus not routinely incorporating it into thyroid function assessments (Health, UCLA, 2023).

I often observe that my clients' blood test results include measurements of free T4 and free T3. It seems that doctors who concentrate on thyroid health typically test for these free hormones. Given their frequent presence in thyroid blood tests, I have decided to include them in the "Thyroid Blood Tests Table" at the end of this chapter.

Benedicte Mai Lerche MSc PhD

Dr. Peat's Thyroid Blood Tests

Some doctors choose to measure just TSH and T4 when assessing a patient's thyroid function. These blood tests are good and informative; however, according to Dr. Ray Peat, they don't make much sense if T3 is not also measured (Peat, 2000, pp. 2-3).

Dr. Peat stated that total T3 can be measured with reasonable accuracy and this single test often correlates better with the metabolic rate than other blood tests (Peat, 2000, p. 2).

He advises evaluating both TSH, total T4, and total T3 as key indicators of thyroid health (Peat, 2000, p. 3).

As previously mentioned, Dr. Peat advocated for a TSH level below 1. Regarding the optimal levels for T4 and T3, many thyroid specialists agree that the most functional, or optimal, levels for both are typically found towards the higher end of the normal range (Wentz, 2023b; Wentz, 2023a; Rupa Health, 2023).

For clarity and to provide a practical guide, specific values will be included in the "Thyroid Blood Tests Table" at the end of this chapter.

In addition to testing for TSH, total T3, and total T4, further valuable information can be obtained by testing for reverse T3 (rT3) and thyroid antibodies. These topics will be explored in the subsequent sections of this chapter.

Ratio of T3 to rT3

As discussed in Chapter 2, levels of reverse T3 (rT3) often rise during situations of crisis, illness, or stress (Alan Jacobs, 2023; Ray Peat Clips, 2016a).

Dr. Ray Peat emphasized that since rT3 acts as an inhibitor to T3, accurately determining the metabolic effects of T3 is not possible without also assessing the rT3 level (Peat, 2008, p. 6; Ray Peat Clips, 2016a).

Therefore, measuring the concentration of rT3 becomes meaningful (Ray Peat Clips, 2016a). A normal level is considered to be between 8-24 ng/dL (Mary Shomon, 2022). However, many thyroid specialists suggest that an optimal rT3 level should be at the lower end of this range. (Stop the thyroid Madness, 2023).

The T3 to rT3 ratio (T3/rT3) is useful in estimating the effective amount of T3 in the body. Ideally, this ratio should exceed 10, indicating significantly more T3 than rT3 in the blood (Alan Jacobs, 2023; Ray Peat Clips, 2016a).
Importantly, if you wish to calculate your T3 to rT3 ratio, it's essential to ensure that the values are in the same units.

While the rT3 blood test is not commonly administered due to ongoing debate over its role in thyroid function assessment (Mary Shomon, 2022; Mary Shomon, 2023b), Dr. Ray Peat considered the rT3 test valuable (Ray Peat Clips, 2016a).

If you have the opportunity to have the rT3 blood test, it can offer useful insights into the state of your thyroid function.

Thyroid Antibody Levels

As outlined in Chapter 2, Hashimoto's thyroiditis is an autoimmune form of hypothyroidism (Very Well Health , 2023b). In Hashimoto's, about 80 to 95 percent of patients have elevated thyroid antibodies (Wentz, 2023b).

The most common antibodies in Hashimoto's thyroiditis are thyroid peroxidase antibodies, typically abbreviated as Anti-TPO or TPOAb, and thyroglobulin antibodies, usually abbreviated as TgAb (Harvard medical School, 2019; Very Well Health , 2023b).

If you have symptoms of hypothyroidism, a healthcare provider can order blood tests to evaluate if you have elevated thyroid antibodies (Very Well Health , 2023b).

When thyroid antibodies fall below 35 IU/mL, they are generally deemed normal by conventional medical criteria (Wentz, 2023b).

Nevertheless, there is some debate among researchers regarding optimal levels. Some suggest that thyroid peroxidase antibodies (anti-TPO, TPOAb) should be under 9 IU/mL and thyroglobulin antibodies (TgAb) below 4 IU/mL (Very Well Health , 2023b). Other researchers argue for even lower thresholds, advocating that the ideal levels for these antibodies should be below 2 IU/mL (Wentz, 2023b).

Some clinicians say that once you have thyroid antibodies, you will always have them (Wentz, 2023b).

As mentioned, Dr. Ray Peat offered a distinctive interpretation of thyroid antibodies, challenging the prevailing medical consensus. He viewed them not as a cause of disorder, but as a signal that the body's repair systems are actively trying to heal the thyroid gland (Ray Peat KMUD, 2013).

Dr. Peat interpreted the presence of thyroid antibodies as an indication that the thyroid gland is under stress (Ray Peat KMUD, 2013). He suggested that this calls for intervention to support thyroid function, which can subsequently lead to a reduction in antibody levels (Ray Peat KMUD, 2013).

It's crucial to note that a diagnosis of Hashimoto's thyroiditis isn't solely based on the presence of thyroid antibodies. Individuals with this condition usually have other blood test indicators of hypothyroidism, such as elevated TSH levels and low T3 and T4 levels (Very Well Health, 2023b).

Additionally, treatment for Hashimoto's thyroiditis is not determined by antibody levels alone but focuses on symptoms and levels of TSH, T4, and T3 hormones (Very Well Health, 2023b). (Wentz, 2023a; Wentz, 2023b).

Benedicte Mai Lerche MSc PhD

Biotin and Blood Test

Biotin, a water-soluble B vitamin commonly used for hair and nail growth, and often present in B-complex supplements, can interfere with thyroid function tests, leading to inaccurate results (American Thyroid Association, 2023b).

From a balanced diet, you will get around 30 mcg of biotin daily, but supplements sometimes contain much higher doses, often ranging from 5,000 to 10,000 mcg (American Thyroid Association, 2023b).

Biotin supplements can skew the results of thyroid function blood tests, often resulting in falsely elevated levels of T4 and T3 and falsely depressed levels of TSH (American Thyroid Association, 2023b). Such misleading test outcomes could lead to an incorrect diagnosis of hyperthyroidism or the incorrect belief that the thyroid hormone dose is too high (American Thyroid Association, 2023a; American Thyroid Association, 2023b).

The American Thyroid Association (ATA) has advised patients to cease biotin supplementation at least 2 days, while other endocrinologists recommend discontinuing biotin supplements for at least 3 days prior to undergoing a blood test for thyroid function

(American Thyroid Association, 2023b; Health, UCLA, 2023).

The time required to clear your body of biotin supplements likely depends on the dosage you have been using. However, if you have been taking high dosages of biotin, to be on the safe side, I recommend stopping biotin supplementation at least 5 days prior to undergoing thyroid blood testing.

Thyroid Meds and Blood Tests

Blood tests for thyroid function are essential for individuals taking thyroid medications, as they help assess the treatment's efficacy.

I often receive questions about the optimal timing for taking thyroid medication relative to these diagnostic tests. It's important to note that taking your thyroid medication too close to the time of your blood test could skew the results (Bodyworks, 2018).

For example, if you're taking a T4-containing medication at 8 a.m. and have your blood test at 10 a.m., the results could show artificially elevated T4 levels. T4 levels have been found to peak about two hours after taking a T4-containing medication (Wentz, 2023a). This could lead your doctor to unnecessarily reduce your medication dosage, even though your T4 levels may be normal for the rest of the day (Bodyworks, 2018).

The timing of tests is especially crucial if you're on medication that includes T3, such as Natural Desiccated Thyroid (NDT), a synthetic T4/T3 combination, or T3 (liothyronine) (Bodyworks, 2018).

Studies show that TSH levels may be suppressed for up to five hours after taking a T3-containing medication, then begin to increase again, stabilizing at around 13 hours post-dose (Wentz, 2023a). Additionally, T3 levels increase after taking T3-containing medication and typically peak about four hours later (Bodyworks, 2018).

Therefore, if you're taking thyroid medication, it's generally recommended to have your blood drawn in the morning before your daily dose (Bodyworks, 2018). If you're on a T3-containing medication, it's optimal to wait about 13 hours after your last dose before testing (Wentz, 2023a).

These precautions help prevent artificially elevated readings of T4 and T3 levels, as well as misleadingly low TSH levels. By doing so, they ensure more accurate lab results, thereby reducing the risk of a false diagnosis of thyroid overdose (Bodyworks, 2018).

For those seeking to measure their body's natural thyroid function without the influence of medication, understanding the half-life of thyroid hormones is crucial. The half-life (T½) refers to the time it takes for the active component of a drug to reduce by 50% in the body.

The half-life of thyroid hormones varies: T4's half-life ranges from 5 to 9 days, meaning it could take up to 9 days for half of the medication to clear from your body (Dansk Endokrinologisk Selskab, 2020; Bodyworks, 2018), while T3's half-life is shorter, ranging from 18 hours to 3 days. It is important to understand that the exact half-life of thyroid hormones varies among individuals (Bodyworks, 2018; Wentz, 2023a).

Figure 4 displays a plot charting the decay time of thyroid hormones in the body. Assuming a half-life of 9 days for T4 and 3 days for T3, it's evident that it can take up to 15 days for T3 to be fully eliminated from the body, and a at least a month for T4.

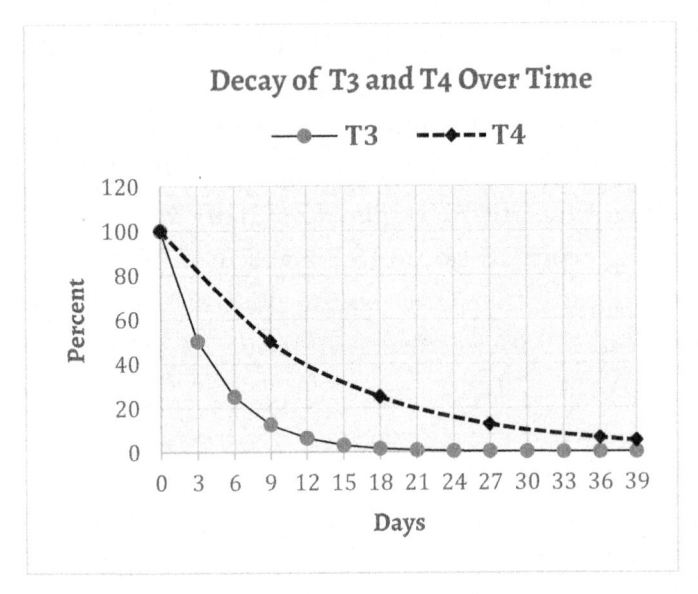

Figure 4: Curves showing the decay time of thyroid hormones in the body, assuming a half-life of 9 days for T4 and 3 days for T3. The plot illustrates the percentage of T4 and T3 remaining in your body as a function of the number of days after stopping the medication.

Thyroid Blood Test Summary

This section offers a brief overview of the key aspects of thyroid blood tests that have been discussed in this chapter.

Dr. Peat's research emphasizes the importance of blood tests for TSH, total T4, total T3, rT3, and thyroid antibodies in evaluating thyroid function.

Key takeaways from Dr. Peat's research include:

TSH Levels: Optimal TSH is below 1 mIU/ml, and levels above 2 mIU/ml are considered high. Hypothyroidism can still occur with a TSH under 1 due to non-thyroidal factors like stress, which can suppress the TSH level.

Total T4: It is advisable to aim for a T4 value in the middle to upper normal range. While many clinicians mainly concentrate on TSH and T4 tests for thyroid function assessment, it's essential to acknowledge that normal levels of these hormones do not necessarily exclude hypothyroidism. This is because some people may not efficiently convert T4 to T3. Therefore, including the T3 test in the evaluation is crucial.

Total T3: Dr. Ray Peat emphasized the importance of the total T3 test. Targeting T3 levels in the middle to upper normal range is advisable. However, it's crucial to understand that optimal T3 levels might not always reflect an effective metabolic rate, since factors such as a diet high in polyunsaturated fats and stress can inhibit the cellular impact of T3.

Reverse T3: The reverse T3 (rT3) test, while not commonly performed, is emphasized by Dr. Ray Peat for its importance. Ideal rT3 levels should be as low as possible or at the lower end of the normal range. The ratio of T3 to rT3 should be greater than 10, indicating that the level of T3 should be at least ten times higher than that of rT3.

Thyroid Antibodies: Dr. Ray Peat considered the presence of thyroid antibodies not as a direct cause of Hashimoto's thyroiditis, but as an indicator that the body's repair mechanisms are active and working to improve thyroid function. It is advised to maintain low levels of thyroid antibodies.

It's crucial to emphasize that there's no specific single optimal number for a given test, as each test result gains significance only when viewed in relation to the other test results, highlighting the importance of a comprehensive analysis of all thyroid blood tests.

The next section features a "Thyroid Blood Tests Table" to help interpret your blood test results. This Table outlines both normal and optimal ranges for these tests.

Benedicte Mai Lerche MSc PhD

Thyroid Blood Tests Table

Table 2 below outlines both standard reference ranges and the optimal or functional ranges for thyroid function blood tests for adults: (Rupa Health, 2023; Sundhed.dk, 2023; Health, UCLA, 2023; Very Well Health, 2023a; Very Well Health , 2023b; Wentz, 2023b; Wentz, 2023a; Clinic, Cleveland, 2022b).

Since laboratories use varying units of measurement, the table displays the same tests in multiple units for comparison.

Be aware that standard reference ranges can vary from one lab to another, which means the ranges on your individual lab report may not correspond exactly to those in the table.

Healthcare providers generally regard results within the standard reference ranges as normal (Very Well Health, 2023a).

Nevertheless, aiming for the optimal ranges is recommended, as these are considered indicative of ideal thyroid function. Please note that these functional ranges are based on research from Dr. Ray Peat and other sources, which may be considered controversial and may not be universally recognized by all healthcare professionals.

Test	Standard Range	Optimal Range
TSH	0.30-5.0 mIU/L	Below 1 mIU/L
Total T4	5-12 µg/dL 65-155 nmol/L	8.5-12 µg/dL 100-155 nmol/L.
Total T3	0,8-2,2 ng/mL 80-220 ng/dL 1,2-3,4 nmol/L	1-2,2 ng/mL 120-220 ng/dL 1.80-3,4 nmol/L
Free T4	7-19 pg/ml 0,7-1,9 ng/dL 9-25 pmol/L	10-19 pg/ml 1-1,9 ng/dL 15-25 pmol/L
Free T3	2,6-4,6 pg/ml 4-7 pmol/L	3-4,6 pg/ml 5-7 pmol/L
Reverse T3	8-24 ng/dL 80-240 pg/mL	Less than 10 ng/dl Less than 100 pg/mL
TPO Ab	Below 35 IU/ml	Below 2IU/ml
TG Ab	Below 35 IU/ml	Below 2IU/ml

Table 2: *Standard and optimal ranges for thyroid function blood tests, values shown for adults.*

Benedicte Mai Lerche MSc PhD

Benedicte Mai Lerche MSc PhD

Chapter 4: At-Home Thyroid Testing

Benedicte Mai Lerche MSc PhD

Comprehensive Testing

Thyroid blood tests primarily measure hormone levels in the blood, but they don't directly assess how these hormones affect cellular functions (Peat, 2001a, p. 72; Wilson, 2015, p. 28).

Dr. Ray Peat highlighted that the presence of active thyroid hormone T3 in the blood doesn't always accurately reflect thyroid function. Factors like unsaturated fats can inhibit how tissues respond to T3 (Peat, 2001a, p. 72).

Dr. Peat also suggested that an effective gauge of thyroid function at the cellular level can be achieved by measuring body temperature and resting pulse rate (Peat, 2001a, p. 72).

Dr. Peat's approach to evaluating thyroid function was comprehensive, integrating blood test results with analyses of pulse and temperature, alongside a thorough evaluation of symptoms (Peat, 2008, pp. 1-6).

In my consultations, I adopt this all-encompassing approach. The remainder of this chapter will concentrate on using pulse and temperature measurements to assess thyroid function.

Benedicte Mai Lerche MSc PhD

Body Temperature

Dr. Ray Peat identified body temperature as a crucial indicator of thyroid function (Peat, 2001a, p. 72), with low body temperature being a well-recognized symptom of hypothyroidism (Wilson, 2015, pp. 24-28; Barnes & Galton, 1976, pp. 42-50).

Renowned American physician Broda Barnes, an expert in hypothyroidism, asserted that measuring basal body temperature upon waking—before leaving the bed—is an effective way to assess thyroid function. Basal body temperature differs from regular body temperature in that it is taken when the body is fully at rest (Barnes & Galton, 1976, p. 5).

Dr. Barnes suggested that patients measure their basal body temperature first thing in the morning, immediately after waking up. This should be done while they are still lying in bed and remaining still, with a thermometer placed under their armpit for ten minutes (Barnes & Galton, 1976, p. 43).

Dr. Ray Peat viewed basal armpit temperature as a reliable indicator of thyroid function. However, he observed that those with hypothyroidism might require several hours for their armpit temperature to stabilize due to their tissues' slowed metabolism. This delay can hinder the quick and accurate measurement of core body temperature through armpit readings in individuals with hypothyroidism (Ray Peat KMUD, 2013).

Dr. Ray Peat recommended assessing thyroid function by measuring the body's temperature orally or using an eardrum thermometer. He advised taking temperature readings first thing in the morning before getting out of bed, again after breakfast, and once more in the afternoon (Peat, 2008, p. 5).

According to Peat, optimal thyroid function is indicated by an oral temperature of around 98°F (36.7°C) upon waking, which should rise to 98.6°F (37°C) after breakfast and remain elevated throughout the day (Peat, 2008, p. 5; Peat, 2001a, p. 72).

The standard adult oral temperature has for many years and is still generally accepted to be around 98.6°F (37°C). It is also generally recognized that the temperature fluctuates over the course of the day with the temperature being lowest in the morning and higher as the day progresses (Illinois Department of Public Health, 2023).

It's essential to recognize that body temperature readings vary based on the method of measurement, as shown in Figure 5 (PeacheHealth, 2022):

- A rectal temperature reading is often 0.5°F (0.3°C) to 1°F (0.6°C) higher compared to an oral temperature.
- An ear (tympanic) temperature reading is usually 0.5°F (0.3°C) to 1°F (0.6°C) above an oral temperature.
- An armpit (axillary) temperature reading is commonly 0.5°F (0.3°C) to 1°F (0.6°C) below an oral temperature.

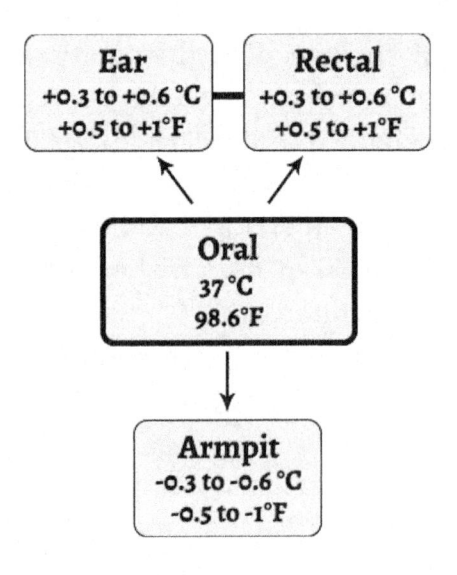

```
┌─────────────────┐   ┌─────────────────┐
│      Ear        │   │     Rectal      │
│  +0.3 to +0.6 °C├───┤  +0.3 to +0.6 °C│
│  +0.5 to +1°F   │   │  +0.5 to +1°F   │
└────────┬────────┘   └────────┬────────┘
         ↖                     ↗
         ┌─────────────────┐
         │      Oral       │
         │     37 °C       │
         │    98.6°F       │
         └────────┬────────┘
                  ↓
         ┌─────────────────┐
         │     Armpit      │
         │  -0.3 to -0.6 °C│
         │  -0.5 to -1°F   │
         └─────────────────┘
```

Figure 5: Depicts the variations in body temperature readings based on different measurement methods.

You can measure your body temperature using rectal, oral, ear, or armpit methods. The rectal method is usually the most accurate, and as previously noted, the armpit method may take longer to yield a stable reading.

Dr. Ray Peat specifically recommended using oral or eardrum measurements for a balance of convenience and accuracy.

The following Table 3 displays typical oral and eardrum temperatures for an adult with optimal thyroid function.

	Fahrenheit	Celsius
Upon waking		
Oral	98 °F	36.7 °C
Ear	99°F	37.2 °C
During the Day		
Oral	98.6 °F	37 °C
Ear	99.6 °F	37.6 °C

Table 3: Body temperature for an adult with good thyroid function according to Dr. Ray Peat.

It's important to recognize that minor deviations from the temperatures outlined are normal, and individual readings may slightly vary from the values in the reference table.

For men and non-menstruating women, consistent body temperature measurements can be taken throughout the month. In contrast, menstruating women experience hormonal fluctuations that can affect body temperature, as noted by Barnes & Galton (Barnes & Galton, 1976, pp. 47-48).

Specifically, the hormone progesterone, produced by the corpus luteum after ovulation, causes a slight rise in a woman's body temperature during the luteal phase—usually by about 0.5-1 degrees Fahrenheit (0.3-0.6 degrees Celsius) (Clearblue, 2023).

In a typical 28-day menstrual cycle, with the first day of menstruation considered day one, ovulation typically occurs around day 15. The temperature will increase right after ovulation and stay elevated until the onset of menstruation, at which point it drops back to the baseline level (Clearblue, 2023).

Dr. Barnes noted that menstruating women should measure their body temperature on the second or third days of their menstrual cycle after flow starts to obtain a more precise baseline (Barnes & Galton, 1976, pp. 47-48).

According to Dr. Ray Peat monitoring body temperature for a minimum of two weeks offers a comprehensive insight into its variations (Peat, 2000, pp. 6-7). It then becomes crucial to account for the effects of progesterone on body temperature and to avoid limiting measurements to the luteal phase, when temperatures are naturally elevated.

Broda Barnes, practicing in the cooler climate of Fort Collins, Colorado, observed that body temperature is an excellent indicator of thyroid function in such conditions (Peat, 2008, p. 4).

However, Dr. Peat noted that in Eugene, Oregon's warm and humid summers, some individuals with clear symptoms of hypothyroidism still had normal body temperatures (Peat, 2008, p. 4).

Dr. Peat emphasized that maintaining a body temperature of 98.6 degrees Fahrenheit (37 degrees Celsius) involves minimal metabolic effort when the external temperature reaches the nineties in Fahrenheit (approximately 32-37 degrees Celsius) (Peat, 2008, p. 4).

Furthermore, individuals in colder climates sleeping under electric blankets may find their morning body temperature artificially elevate (Peat, 2008, p. 4).

Dr. Peat concluded that in conditions such as hot, humid weather, or when using an electric blanket, body temperature alone may not be a reliable measure of thyroid function. He advocated for a comprehensive approach that evaluates both body temperature and pulse rate to assess thyroid health thoroughly (Peat, 2008, p. 4).

The subsequent section will focus on the significance of pulse rate as a metric for thyroid function assessment.

Pulse Rate

Dr. Ray Peat considered the resting pulse rate a vital indicator of thyroid function (Peat, 2008, p. 4). A low resting pulse rate is recognized as a sign of hypothyroidism (Harward Medical School, 2023; Bhatt, 2020).

The terms 'resting pulse rate' and 'resting heart rate' are interchangeably used to describe the number of heart beats per minute when the body is at rest (Mayo Clinic, 2022a; British Heart Foundation, 2021).

The heart's role is to pump blood, delivering oxygen to the body's tissues—a critical function of the circulatory system (Howard E. LeWine, 2023).

A healthy heart doesn't operate with clock-like regularity but adjusts its rhythm to meet changing oxygen demands throughout the day (Howard E. LeWine, 2023). At rest, the body's demand for oxygen is at its lowest, and the heart circulates just enough blood to meet this minimal requirement, allowing for an accurate measurement of the resting pulse rate (Howard E. LeWine, 2023).

The normal resting pulse rate for adults is officially considered to range from 60 to 100 beats per minute (Mayo Clinic, 2022a; Howard E. LeWine, 2023).

The common belief is that a lower resting pulse rate is indicative of good health, a view often supported by medical and fitness experts. However, it's crucial to understand the specific causes behind a low resting pulse rate.

Endurance athletes typically exhibit resting pulse rates lower than the average (Oh, 2016; Mayo Clinic, 2022a).

Regular physical activity, particularly of vigorous intensity, strengthens the heart muscle. This enhanced conditioning allows the heart to pump more blood with each beat (National heart, lung and blood institute, 2022). As a result, the heart of a physically fit individual doesn't need to beat as frequently to distribute oxygen effectively throughout the body, leading to lower resting pulse rates in athletes (Bhatt, 2020; Oh, 2016).
However, it's important to note that a low resting pulse doesn't universally signify good health. For those who are not athletes or don't engage regularly in high-intensity physical activities, a low resting pulse might be a sign of hypothyroidism (Bhatt, 2020; Peat, 2001d, p. 17).

A resting pulse rate below 60 beats per minute is considered low and is medically termed as bradycardia (British Heart Foundation, 2021). Bradycardia can be problematic if the heart is unable to pump sufficient oxygen-rich blood (Mayo Clinic, 2022b).

Dr. Ray Peat found that, while the medical community often considers a resting pulse rate as low as 60 beats per minute normal for non-athletes, such a low pulse could indicate hypothyroidism (Peat, 2001d, p. 104). He noted that healthy individuals with good thyroid function usually have an average resting pulse rate of about 85 beats per minute, whereas those in less-than-optimal health often have rates around 70 beats per minute (Peat, 2008, p. 4).

Typically, it is normal to wake up with a lower pulse rate, which then increases to 80 - 90 beats per minute after breakfast and remains elevated throughout the day (Table 4) (Peat, 2008, p. 5; Ray Peat Clips, 2016d; Functional Performance, 2023).

	Beats per minute
Upon waking	75-80
During the Day	80-90

Table 4: *Resting pulse rate for an adult with good thyroid function according to Dr. Ray Peat.*

It's essential to understand that heart rate can be influenced by a variety of factors (British Heart Foundation, 2021).

Medications play a significant role: for instance, asthma medications might increase pulse rate, while beta blockers often have a lowering effect. Other factors that can affect heart rate include illnesses, fever, smoking, anxiety, and specific health conditions such as heart disease (British Heart Foundation, 2021; Mayo Clinic, 2022a).

Furthermore, it's crucial to recognize that not all individuals with hypothyroidism present with low pulse rates and body temperatures. In fact, elevated levels of stress hormones, commonly associated with hypothyroidism, can lead to an increase in both resting pulse rate and body temperature. This aspect will be delved into in greater detail in the following section.

Effect of Stress Hormones

Understanding that individuals with low thyroid function often compensate by producing higher levels of stress hormones, such as cortisol and adrenaline, is crucial (Peat, 2008, pp. 4-5; Peat, 2001a, p. 72). These hormones can significantly alter a person's appearance and physiological markers, potentially misleading healthcare professionals (Peat, 2008, p. 6).

Understanding the complex interplay between thyroid function and stress hormones is crucial. Elevated cortisol levels, for instance, are commonly observed in individuals with hypothyroidism. These elevated levels not only help maintain body temperature but can also induce a catabolic state in some cases. In this state, the body breaks down both fat and muscle, leading to an overall loss of body mass (Peat, 2008, pp. 5-6; Healthline, 2019).

In cases of hypothyroidism, a lower pulse rate can sometimes be attributed to insufficient compensatory production of adrenaline (Peat, 2008, p. 5). Dr. Ray Peat noted that many individuals with hypothyroidism exhibit adrenaline levels up to 40 times higher than average, which can cause circulatory issues like an elevated pulse rate and high blood pressure, further complicating the clinical picture (Peat, 2001a, p. 72; Peat, 2008, p. 6).

When a very thin person presents with high blood pressure and a high pulse rate, doctors may not immediately consider hypothyroidism. This possibility can be overlooked despite elevated TSH levels and low T4 and T3, often because of common medical stereotypes. Furthermore, if these test results are within the normal range, the individual risks being misdiagnosed with hyperthyroidism (Peat, 2008, p. 6).

It is imperative for healthcare providers to recognize the common adaptive reactions to thyroid deficiency, such as the catabolic effects induced by elevated cortisol and the circulatory disturbances from high adrenaline (Peat, 2008, p. 6). Acknowledging these factors should encourage more targeted testing, which is vital for an accurate diagnosis and effective treatment of hypothyroidism (Peat, 2008, p. 6).

Understanding that cortisol and adrenaline significantly impact pulse and temperature readings is crucial, as this complicates the use of these metrics as indicators of thyroid function (Peat, 2008, p. 5).

Typically, adrenaline and cortisol levels begin to rise after a person goes to bed. For those with hypothyroidism, these levels can spike sharply, with adrenaline peaking around 1 or 2 A.M., and cortisol around dawn (Peat, 2008, p. 5). It's not uncommon for people to wake up with a pounding heart during the adrenaline surge (Peat, 2008, p. 5).

A person with hypothyroidism often experiences heightened stress at night, leading to increased levels of stress hormones. These elevated stress hormones can persist throughout the night and into the morning. While adrenaline tends to raise both pulse and temperature, cortisol mainly increases temperature (Peat, 2008, p. 5).

Measuring pulse and temperature upon waking and assuming these metrics accurately reflect thyroid function can be misleading due to the influence of stress hormones (Peat, 2008, p. 5).
After consuming a balanced breakfast cortisol and adrenaline levels typically begin to normalize as blood sugar is sustained by food, instead of the stress hormones. This is an opportune time to measure both temperature and pulse rate, as it offers a clearer indication of thyroid function, free from the distortive effects of stress hormones (Peat, 2008, p. 5; Ray Peat KMUD, 2013).

While temperature and pulse rate typically rise after a balanced breakfast in healthy individuals, those with hypothyroidism may experience a decrease in one or both of these measurements (Peat, 2008, p. 5; Ray Peat KMUD, 2013).

Dr. Ray Peat underlines the necessity of incorporating both carbohydrates and proteins in a balanced breakfast. This combination helps elevate blood sugar and decrease stress hormones (Peat, 2008, p. 5).

A balanced breakfast could feature butter-fried eggs, generously seasoned with salt, accompanied by carbohydrate-rich fruits such as orange juice. Alternatively, one could opt for salty cheese or Greek yogurt paired with fruit. Including salt in a balanced breakfast, such as adding a pinch of salt to your orange juice, can be beneficial, as salt is known to lower adrenaline levels (Peat, 2001a, p. 79).

While coffee is generally part of Dr. Ray Peat's dietary guidelines and certainly a staple in his own breakfast routine, it's important to be aware that many people with hypothyroidism may experience a stress reaction to caffeine. For individuals with hypothyroidism, being mindful of their body's reactions is crucial. Symptoms such as increased pulse rates and jitteriness after drinking coffee can indicate an adrenaline-like response to caffeine (Peat, 2001d, pp. 76-77). In such cases, avoiding coffee might be wise to prevent any adverse effects on pulse and temperature readings.

Measuring temperature and pulse rate upon waking, and approximately 30-40 minutes after a balanced breakfast, is recommended. This practice can help differentiate the effects of stress hormones from those related to thyroid function. Taking temperature and pulse measurements again in the afternoon provides further valuable insight into thyroid health (Peat, 2008, p. 5).

It is important to mention that you can take multiple readings of temperature and pulse throughout the day. Focusing on pre- and post-meal measurements can help distinguish the effects of thyroid function from stress, as cortisol and adrenaline levels normally come down after a meal.

Benedicte Mai Lerche MSc PhD

Measuring Temperature

For measuring body temperature, Dr. Ray Peat recommended measuring either the oral or eardrum temperature, using either a digital oral or digital eardrum thermometer.

Although basal digital thermometers that measure oral temperature to two decimal places are available, Dr. Peat suggested that such precision is not necessary for thyroid function assessment. He recommended using just a standard digital thermometer for measuring oral temperature (Ray Peat KMUD, 2013).

My personal preference leans towards the digital eardrum thermometer, because it is not affected by recent consumption of hot or cold beverages or tooth brushing, which can alter oral temperature readings. Additionally, eardrum thermometers are notably fast, delivering a reading within seconds.

Keep in mind that temperatures measured at the eardrum are typically slightly higher than oral readings. An eardrum temperature reading is approximately 0.5°F (0.3°C) to 1°F (0.6°C) higher than an oral reading.

Here are instructions for measuring oral and eardrum temperatures (Mayo Clinic, 2020).

For oral temperature measurement:

1. Wait for 30 minutes after eating or drinking before taking an oral temperature.
2. Turn on the thermometer and place it under your tongue.
3. Keep your mouth closed and wait until the thermometer beeps, indicating that the measurement is complete.
4. Read the temperature from the display.

For ear temperature measurements:

1. Ensure that your ear canal is dry before measuring.
2. Turn on the thermometer and insert it into the ear canal, following the instructions provided.
3. Wait for the beep, which signals the end of the measurement.
4. Read the temperature.

Avoid measuring temperature immediately after physical activity or exposure to heat. For accuracy, rest for five minutes before taking your measurement.

Measuring Pulse Rate

To my knowledge, Dr. Ray Peat didn't advise on any specific way to measure the resting pulse rate.

Personally, I use a digital/automated blood pressure monitor to check my pulse rate, which provides both pulse and blood pressure readings at the same time.

You can also measure your pulse at your wrist or neck. Below are the instructions for how to do this (Harvard Medical School, 2021):

For wrist and neck pulse measurements:

1. To check your pulse at the wrist, place your index and middle fingers lightly on the opposite wrist, just below the base of your thumb.
2. For neck measurements, place your fingers gently to the side under your jawbone.
3. Then count the beats for either 30 seconds and multiply by two, or 15 seconds and multiply by four, to calculate your beats per minute.

For the most accurate reading, take your pulse while you are calm and rested, not immediately following physical exertion or a stressful occurrence, as these can raise your heart rate temporarily. For optimal results, sit quietly for five minutes before measuring your resting pulse rate (Harvard Medical School, 2021).

A Note on Wearables

Many clients are curious about using wearable devices such as smartwatches, smart rings, or fitness trackers to monitor their pulse rate and body temperature.

It's important to understand that when wearable devices measure temperature, they are actually measuring skin temperature, which is different from core body temperature. Skin temperature can be influenced by environmental factors, making it less accurate for precise measurements like those needed for assessing thyroid function. This is why traditional methods of measuring body temperature, as previously discussed in this chapter, are generally more reliable (Wearables, 2022).

While wearable devices are effective at detecting temperature changes — useful for signaling events such as ovulation or the onset of illness (Wearables, 2022) — they should not, in my opinion, replace oral or eardrum temperature measurements for thyroid function assessment.

Monitoring heart rate is more straightforward with wearable devices. Many of these devices can accurately monitor resting pulse rates (Cleveland Clinic, 2022a).

However, for superior performance, chest-band devices are recommended. These use electrical detection to measure the heart rate directly, ensuring exceptional accuracy whether you're at rest or engaging in activities like running or cycling (Harvard Medical School, 2021).

For measuring pulse rate, wearable devices worn on the wrist or forearm, such as smartwatches, usually provide accurate readings when you are at rest. Smart rings are reported to offer the same level of precision, as noted by the Cleveland Clinic (Cleveland Clinic, 2022a).

To verify the accuracy of these wearable devices in measuring your resting pulse rate, comparing their readings with those from a manual pulse check or a digital blood pressure monitor is advisable.

Pulse and Temp Summary

Both low body temperature and reduced pulse rate are established indicators of hypothyroidism (Wilson, 2015, pp. 24-28; Barnes & Galton, 1976, p. 285; Bhatt, 2020).

Dr. Ray Peat recommended using these metrics together to evaluate thyroid function, as they provide insights into cellular metabolism (Peat, 2001a, p. 72; Ray Peat KMUD, 2013; Ray Peat Clips, 2016e, p. 76; Peat, 2008, p. 5).

Dr. Peat suggested taking temperature and pulse readings immediately after waking up, then again 30-40 minutes following a balanced breakfast, and once more in the afternoon (Peat, 2008, p. 5; Functional Performance, 2023).

According to Dr. Ray Peat, optimal thyroid function is indicated by an initial waking oral temperature of approximately 98°F (36.7°C), which should rise to about 98.6°F (37°C) after breakfast and remain at this level throughout the day. Additionally, an ideal resting pulse rate is around 85 beats per minute (Ray Peat Clips, 2016d; Peat, 2001b, p. 76; Peat, 2008, p. 4).

People with hypothyroidism often have oral temperatures and pulse rates significantly below these values (Peat, 2001d, p. 17).

It's important to note that individuals with hypothyroidism may produce more stress hormones, potentially raising both pulse and temperature.

Comparing pre- and post-breakfast measurements helps distinguish between the effects of stress hormones and actual thyroid function (Peat, 2008, p. 5).

A drop in pulse and/or temperature after breakfast suggests elevated stress hormones, with post-meal readings being more indicative of true thyroid function (Peat, 2008, p. 5).

Dr. Peat's method of evaluating thyroid function using pulse and temperature, as well as symptom evaluation, enables proactive, non-intrusive monitoring of thyroid health at home. This approach is essential when assessing metabolic health. Additionally, it is crucial for people on thyroid medication, where regular monitoring of pulse, temperature, and symptoms is vital. Daily readings initially help determine the correct dosage. Once stable, continued tracking assesses medication effectiveness and can signal when further thyroid tests might optimize treatment. I am planning to write a future book in the "Healing Metabolism" series, focusing on Dr. Ray Peat's thyroid medication protocol.

Benedicte Mai Lerche MSc PhD

Pulse and Temp Table

In Table 5 below temperature and pulse rate for an adult with good thyroid function is summarized.

It's completely normal for measurements to vary slightly from the values presented. However, if you consistently have a low body temperature and reduced pulse rate, coupled with various hypothyroidism symptoms, it strongly suggests low thyroid function. This diagnosis can be further confirmed with thyroid blood tests (Peat, 2001b, p. 76).

In the following section, I will provide schemas for pulse and temperature tracking, including a 14-day tracking template. These resources will aid in consistently monitoring your pulse and temperature. Additionally, you will find a questionnaire designed to help identify symptoms of hypothyroidism.

Body Temperature		
	Fahrenheit	Celsius
Upon waking		
Oral	98 °F	36.7 °C
Ear	99 °F	37.2 °C
During the Day		
Oral	98.6 °F	37 °C
Ear	99.6 °F	37.6 °C

Pulse rate		
	Beats/minute	
Upon waking	75-80	
During the Day	80-90	

Table 5: Pulse and temperature for an adult with good thyroid function according to Dr. Ray Peat.

Benedicte Mai Lerche MSc PhD

Chapter 5: Track your Thyroid Function

Benedicte Mai Lerche MSc PhD

Pulse, Temp, Symptoms Logs

The schemas below outline a structured approach for monitoring physiological markers indicative of low thyroid function.

Schema 1 illustrates how to maintain a daily log for recording pulse and body temperature. Taking multiple readings to calculate an average can provide a more accurate assessment of your metabolic rate.

Schema 2 is designed for a bi-weekly overview, facilitating the transfer of average values from your daily logs to track trends over time. Don't worry about missing some entries; the overall pattern is most important.

Schema 3, developed from the common symptoms of hypothyroidism detailed in Chapter 2, provides a checklist for recording the symptoms you experience. Noting any additional symptoms, you encounter will offer further insight into the severity of your hypothyroidism. By correlating pulse, temperature, and symptoms with blood test results for thyroid function, you can evaluate your metabolic health.

These metrics can be useful for discussions with your healthcare provider to gain insights into your thyroid function. Additionally, I offer counseling sessions where we can review these metrics together. You can schedule a session at biochemnordic.com.

Shema 1: *Daily log for pulse and temperature*

Date:	Temp	Pulse
Before breakfast	1 2 3 ------------------ Avg:	1 2 3 ------------------ Avg:
After breakfast	1 2 3 ------------------ Avg:	1 2 3 ------------------ Avg:
Afternoon/ Evening	1 2 3 ------------------ Avg:	1 2 3 ------------------ Avg:

Benedicte Mai Lerche MSc PhD

Shema 2: *A biweekly log for pulse and temperature.*

Day	Before breakfast		After breakfast		Afternoon	
	Temp.	Pulse	Temp.	Pulse	Temp.	Pulse
1						
2						
3						
4						
5						
6						
7						
8						
9						
10						
11						
12						
13						
14						

Benedicte Mai Lerche MSc PhD

Shema 3: *Checklist of hypothyroidism symptoms.*

Mark your symptoms:
Fatigue: Feeling tired and lacking energy, even after getting adequate rest (chronic fatigue).
Headaches: Experiencing pressure headaches and migraines.
Hypoglycemia: Having low blood sugar, resulting in a need to eat frequently to avoid feeling faint and dizzy.
Weight changes: Experiencing unexplained weight gain or difficulty losing weight despite maintaining a healthy diet and regular exercise routine. Some individuals may also experience weight loss.
Low body temperature: Having cold intolerance, feeling excessively cold even in warm temperatures, and having cold hands and feet.
Reduced heart rate: Experiencing a slow heart rate (bradycardia) and decreased heart function.
Heart problems & disease: Experiencing heart pain, poor heart sounds, enlargement of the heart, palpitations, and hypertension.
Constipation: Experiencing slow digestion, difficulty passing stools, and infrequent bowel movements.

Digestive problems: Painful digestion, irritable bowel syndrome (IBS), as well as an overgrowth of bad bacteria and candida.
Dry skin: Having dry, rough, thin, pale skin that may be itchy and scaly, accompanied by conditions like eczema or skin infections.
Brittle hair & nails: Experiencing thinning of hair and nails, hair loss, changes in hair texture, and potential loss of the outer third of the eyebrows.
Muscle and joint pain: Experiencing muscle aches, stiffness, and joint pain not attributed to any specific injury or physical activity.
Carpal tunnel syndrome: Having pain, numbness, and tingling sensations in the hand, arms, and fingers (carpal tunnel syndrome).
Mood changes: Experiencing depression, anxiety, irritability, and mood swings.
Cognitive impairment: Having difficulty concentrating, poor memory, and decreased mental alertness (brain fog).
Hoarseness: Experiencing a deepening or hoarse voice, often accompanied by a sore throat.

Swelling: Experiencing water retention (edema), often with swelling or puffiness in the face, hands, feet, or ankles.
High cholesterol: Having elevated levels of cholesterol in the blood, even with a healthy diet and lifestyle.
Decreased libido: Experiencing a loss of interest in sexual activity and a reduced sexual drive.
Menstrual irregularities: Having irregular menstrual cycles, heavy menstrual bleeding, prolonged menstrual periods, painful menstruation, and experiencing symptoms of premenstrual syndrome (PMS) and polycystic ovaries (PCOS).
Infertility & miscarriage: Experiencing male and female infertility, with a higher chance of miscarriage in females.
Insomnia: Having problems falling asleep and/or waking up during the night.
Other symptoms: Poor vision, hearing loss, anemia, allergies, frequent colds, infections, orange calluses, inflammation, premature aging, and more.
Symptoms not listed above:

Benedicte Mai Lerche MSc PhD

Chapter 6: Healing Metabolism

Benedicte Mai Lerche MSc PhD

Benedicte Mai Lerche MSc PhD

Dr. Ray Peat's Health Method

Physicians often rely on blood tests to diagnose thyroid issues. However, as this book indicates, these tests have very large reference ranges, which can result in missed diagnoses of hypothyroidism, despite the presence of symptoms indicating low thyroid function.

If the testing strategies outlined in this book indicate that your health challenges could be linked to suboptimal thyroid function, you may face an urgent question: How can you effectively increase your metabolic rate to restore lost vitality?

My approach to managing low thyroid function is deeply rooted in my personal triumph over hypothyroidism and the groundbreaking research of Dr. Ray Peat.

Adopting Dr. Ray Peat's health principles marked a pivotal moment in my fight against hypothyroidism. His insights were transformative, leading me from battling numerous low thyroid symptoms to achieving vibrant well-being. Without his guidance, I would likely still be confronting health issues today. My steadfast belief in Dr. Peat's approach motivates me to share his principles, aiming to help others overcome their metabolic and hormonal imbalances.

This mission is fulfilled through my book series "Healing Metabolism" and the resources on my website, biochemnordic.com.

In the following, I will outline key aspects of Dr. Ray Peat's health philosophy.

Dr. Peat contends that illnesses often result from an imbalance between the body's energy resources and the demands of its environment. Given the critical role of the active thyroid hormone T3 in regulating cellular energy, maintaining strong thyroid function is crucial for overall well-being. Therefore, it's imperative to adopt a lifestyle that strengthens metabolic health, serving as a foundation for enduring wellness.

A crucial aspect of Dr. Ray Peat's approach to health is the consistent adoption of a diet that supports thyroid function.
Dr. Peat has made significant advances in nutritional science, especially regarding the relationship between diet, hormones, and health. His research has established the foundation for what is now known as the 'Ray Peat diet.' This dietary regimen promotes

food choices that enhance thyroid function and discourage those that inhibit metabolic activity.

Dr. Peat's dietary guidelines notably diverge from conventional nutritional advice. However, the comprehensive biochemical rationale behind each recommendation strongly appeals to those seeking a more scientific approach to the interplay between nutrition and health.

Another key aspect of Dr. Ray Peat's research is the appropriate use of thyroid replacement therapy. Dr. Peat has pointed out that relying exclusively on levothyroxine (T4) for treating hypothyroidism might be insufficient or even problematic for individuals who have difficulty converting T4 into the active thyroid hormone T3. He advocated for a treatment approach that combines T4 and T3 hormones in a ratio that mimics the natural secretion of the human thyroid gland.

Additionally, Dr. Peat's protocol often includes supplements with natural hormones, such as progesterone and pregnenolone. These hormones are known for their anti-estrogenic and anti-stress effects and may be beneficial for a variety of health issues, including hypothyroidism, stress, inflammation, PMS, and infertility. His health strategy also extends to nutritional supplements, digestive aids, and light therapy, among other treatments.

It's important to understand that while following Dr. Peat's health principles can lead to swift healing and symptom relief, his philosophy is fundamentally geared towards a long-term commitment to maintaining optimal metabolic health.

For those interested in gaining a further understanding of Dr. Ray Peat's healing philosophy, my previous book, "How I Overcame Hypothyroidism," is an invaluable resource. It details my health journey and the strategies I employed to overcome hypothyroidism, all under Dr. Peat's guidance.

You are also encouraged to visit my website, biochemnordic.com. There, you'll find a range of online educational materials, and you can book video counseling sessions with me. Additionally, while visiting the site, you have the option to subscribe to my free mailing list, keeping you updated on my latest endeavors and other relevant news.

Your Review Matters

If you found this book valuable, I would be immensely grateful if you could take a moment to leave a review on the platform where you purchased the book or on Goodreads.

Your feedback will help other potential readers facing similar health challenges to discover and benefit from my work.

Just a few thoughtful lines from you can make a significant impact.

Thank you sincerely for your support!

Benedicte Mai Lerche

Benedicte Mai Lerche MSc PhD

About the Author

Benedicte Mai Lerche earned an MSc in Biochemistry from the University of Copenhagen and a Ph.D. in Chemical and Biochemical Engineering from the Technical University of Denmark.

Benedicte is deeply committed to assisting individuals in overcoming challenges associated with low thyroid function and hormonal imbalances.

Through her website, biochemnordic.com, she provides a wealth of e-learning materials and personalized video counseling, aiming to support individuals worldwide on their health journey.

With a primary focus on supporting optimal thyroid function and boosting cellular energy production, Benedicte shares invaluable knowledge on dietary principles, supplement recommendations, and lifestyle factors that promote efficient metabolism and hormone balance, while also offering anti-aging, anti-stress, and anti-inflammatory benefits.

Driven by the profound impact of Dr. Ray Peat's extensive research, Benedicte has personally witnessed the transformative power of his insights in addressing her own thyroid and hormonal struggles. This experience has fueled her dedication to impart Dr. Peat's invaluable knowledge to others who are encountering similar issues.

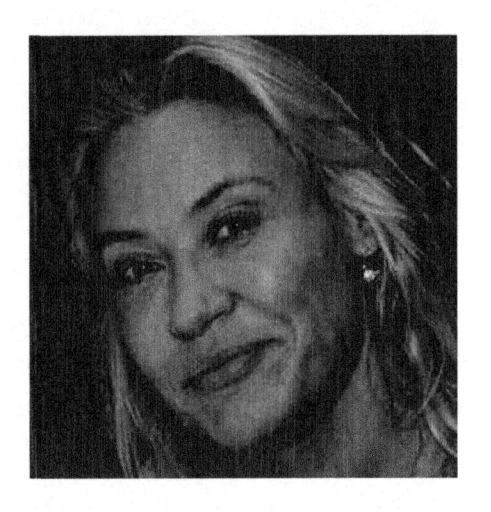

Benedicte Mai Lerche MSc PhD

References

Alan Jacobs, M., 2023. *What is the Reverse T3 Syndrome?*. [Online]
Available at: https://neuroendocrinology.org/what-is-the-reverse-t3-syndrome/#:~:text=It%20is%20known%20that%20the,this%20as%20the%20RT3%20Syndrome.

American Thyroid Association, 2023a. *Thyroid Function Tests.* [Online]
Available at: https://www.thyroid.org/thyroid-function-tests/
[Accessed 22 August 2023].

American Thyroid Association, 2023b. *Thyroid function tests - Biotin supplements.* [Online]
Available at: https://www.thyroid.org/patient-thyroid-information/ct-for-patients/december-2018/vol-11-issue-12-p-3-4/
[Accessed August 2023].

Barnes, B. & Galton, L., 1976. *Hypothyroidism The Unsuspected Illness.* s.l.:HarperCollins.

Bhatt, D. L., 2020. *Havard Health Puplishing*. [Online]
Available at:
https://www.health.harvard.edu/heart-health/is-a-low-heart-rate-worrisome

Bikle, D. D., 2021. The Free Hormone Hypothesis: When, Why, and How to Measure the Free Hormone Levels to Assess Vitamin D, Thyroid, Sex Hormone, and Cortisol Status. *JBMR Plus*.

Bodyworks, 2018. *When To Take Thyroid Medications To Get Accurate Lab Results*. [Online]
Available at:
https://www.askdrrapp.com/blog/40383-timing-your-thyroid-medications-to-get-accurate-lab-results

Boston University School of Public Health, 2017. *Respiratory health*. [Online]
Available at:
https://sphweb.bumc.bu.edu/otlt/MPH-Modules/PH/RespiratoryHealth/

British Heart Foundation, 2021. *HEART MATTERS*. [Online]
Available at:
https://www.bhf.org.uk/informationsupport/heart-matters-magazine/medical/ask-the-experts/pulse-rate#:~:text=Your%20pulse%20rate%2C%20als

o%20known,vary%20from%20minute%20to%20minute.

Clearblue, 2023. *All about the luteal phase.* [Online] Available at: https://www.clearblue.com/menstrual-cycle/luteal-phase

Cleveland Clinic, 2019. *Thyroid Issues? What You Should Know About Foods and Supplements to Avoid.* [Online] Available at: https://health.clevelandclinic.org/thyroid-issues-what-you-need-to-know-about-diet-and-supplements/

Cleveland Clinic, 2022a. *Heart Rate Monitor.* [Online] Available at: https://my.clevelandclinic.org/health/diagnostics/23429-heart-rate-monitor

Cleveland Clinic, 2023. *Hypothyroidism.* [Online] Available at: https://my.clevelandclinic.org/health/diseases/12120-hypothyroidism

Clinic, Cleveland, 2022b. *T3 (Triiodothyronine) Test.* [Online] Available at: https://my.clevelandclinic.org/health/diagnostics/22425-triiodothyronine-t3

Dansk Endokrinologisk Selskab, 2020. *Hypothyroidism.* [Online]
Available at: https://endocrinology.dk/nbv/thyroideasygdomme/hypothyroidisme/

Everyday Health, 2018. *Do You Really Need to Give Up Kale, Cauliflower, and Other Cruciferous Vegetables When You Have Hypothyroidism?.* [Online]
Available at: https://www.everydayhealth.com/hs/hypothyroidism/do-you-need-to-avoid-cruciferous-vegetables/

Faix, J. D., 2013. *Thyroid-Stimulating Hormone | AACC.org.* [Online]
Available at: https://www.aacc.org/cln/articles/2013/may/tsh-harmonization

Functional Performance, 2023. *Temperature and Pulse Basics & Monthly Log.* [Online]
Available at: https://www.functionalps.com/blog/2012/11/19/temperature-and-pulse-basics-monthly-log/

Garnet Health, 2016. *Basal Metabolic Rate Calculator.* [Online]
Available at:

https://www.garnethealth.org/news/basal-metabolic-rate-calculator

Grant, S., 2019. *Understanding your thyroid hormone blood test results.* [Online]
Available at:
https://stevegranthealth.com/articles-posts/understanding-your-thyroid-hormone-blood-test-results/

Harvard medical School, 2019. *Is there a role for surgery in treating Hashimoto's thyroiditis?.* [Online]
Available at:
https://www.health.harvard.edu/blog/is-there-a-role-for-surgery-in-treating-hashimotos-thyroiditis-2019081217443

Harvard Medical School, 2021. *Want to check your heart rate? Here's how.* [Online]
Available at:
https://www.health.harvard.edu/heart-health/want-to-check-your-heart-rate-heres-how

Harward Medical School, 2023. *Thyroid hormone: How it affects your heart.* [Online]
Available at:
https://www.health.harvard.edu/heart-health/thyroid-hormone-how-it-affects-your-heart#:~:text=Hypothyroidism%20can%20affe

ct%20the%20heart,circulate%20blood%20around%20the%20body.

Health Central, 2021. *What Is Reverse T3?*. [Online]
Available at:
https://www.healthcentral.com/condition/thyroid/what-is-reverse-t3

Health, UCLA, 2023. *ENDOCRINE SURGERY: Normal Thyroid Hormone Levels.* [Online]
Available at:
https://www.uclahealth.org/medical-services/surgery/endocrine-surgery/conditions-treated/thyroid/normal-thyroid-hormone-levels#:~:text=TSH%20normal%20values%20are%200.5,0.7%20to%201.9ng%2FdL
[Accessed 10 August 2023].

HealthCentral, K. M. M. M., 2014. *Hashimoto's Thyroiditis Diagnosis.* [Online]
Available at:
https://www.healthcentral.com/condition/hashimotos-thyroiditis/hashimotos-thyroiditis-diagnosis

Healthline, 2019. *Catabolism vs. Anabolism: What's the Difference?.* [Online]
Available at:
https://www.healthline.com/health/catabolism-vs-anabolism#body-weight

Howard E. LeWine, M., 2023. *What is a normal heart rate?*. [Online]
Available at: https://www.health.harvard.edu/heart-health/what-your-heart-rate-is-telling-you

Illinois Department of Public Health, 2023. *Thermometers and Fever.* [Online]
Available at: http://www.idph.state.il.us/public/hb/hbthermometers.htm#:~:text=Average%20body%20temperature%20is%3A,%3A%2099.6F%20(37.5 C)

Mary Shomon, 2022. *Overview of Reverse T3 Thyroid Hormone.* [Online]
Available at: https://www.verywellhealth.com/reverse-t3-thyroid-hormone-overview-3233184#toc-possible-significance

Mary Shomon, 2023a. *Reading Your Thyroid Blood Test Results.* [Online]
Available at: https://www.verywellhealth.com/interpret-your-thyroid-test-results-3231840

Mary Shomon, 2023b. *Leptin, rT3, and Weight Gain With Hypothyroidism.* [Online]
Available at:

https://www.verywellhealth.com/hypothyroidism-leptin-rt3-weight-gain-3233049

Mayo Clinic, 2020. *How to take your temperature?*. [Online]
Available at: https://www.mayoclinic.org/how-to-take-temperature/art-20482578

Mayo Clinic, 2022a. *What's a normal resting heart rate?*. [Online]
Available at: https://www.mayoclinic.org/healthy-lifestyle/fitness/expert-answers/heart-rate/faq-20057979

Mayo Clinic, 2022b. *Bradycardia.* [Online]
Available at: https://www.mayoclinic.org/diseases-conditions/bradycardia/symptoms-causes/syc-20355474

National heart, lung and blood institute, 2022. *PHYSICAL ACTIVITY AND YOUR HEART.* [Online]
Available at: https://www.nhlbi.nih.gov/health/heart/physical-activity/benefits#:~:text=When%20done%20regularly%2C%20moderate%2D%20and,levels%20in%20your%20blood%20rise.

Oh, D. J. H. H. O. &. L. B. A., 2016. The effects of strenuous exercises on resting heart rate, blood pressure, and maximal oxygen uptake.. *Journal of exercise rehabilitation,,* 12(1), p. 42–46..

PeacheHealth, 2022. *Fever Temperatures: Accuracy and Comparison.* [Online] Available at: https://www.peacehealth.org/medical-topics/id/tw9223

Peat, R., 2000. Thyroid: Therapies, Confusion, and Fraud. *Ray Peat's Newsletter,* May.pp. 1-7.

Peat, R., 2001a. *Generative Energy: Restoring the Wholeness of Life.* s.l.:Raymond Peat PhD.

Peat, R., 2001b. *From PMS to Menopause: Female Hormones in Context.* s.l.:Raymond Peat Ph.D..

Peat, R., 2001d. *Nutrition for Women: 100 Short Articles.* s.l.:Raymond Peat Ph.D..

Peat, R., 2008. TSH, temperature, pulse rate, and other indicators in hypothyroidism. *Ray Peat's Newsletter,* January.pp. 2-6.

Pediatric On Call, 2023. *Basal Metabolic Rate (BMR).* [Online] Available at: https://www.pediatriconcall.com/calculators/basel-metabolic-rate-bmr-calculator

Ray Peat Clips, 2016a. *Ray Peat on thyroid labs and T3, T4, rT3, TSH..* [Online]
Available at: https://www.youtube.com/watch?v=HynVEuBiCpM
[Accessed 10 August 2023].

Ray Peat Clips, 2016c. *Ray Peat on TSH levels, inflammation..* [Online]
Available at: https://www.youtube.com/watch?v=v9GqRNO0loc

Ray Peat Clips, 2016d. *Ray Peat on heart rate and benefits of high heart rate. Body temperature..* [Online]
Available at: https://www.youtube.com/watch?v=xJb-2IYXA8w

Ray Peat Clips, 2016e. *Ray Peat on the importance of the liver and liver health.* [Online]
Available at: https://www.youtube.com/watch?v=wxTwBY5r_qA

Ray Peat Clips, 2021. *Ray Peat on Dosing T3.* [Online]
Available at: https://www.youtube.com/watch?v=P9A8ap4TU2c

Ray Peat KMUD, 2013. *Hashimoto's, Antibodies, Temperature and Pulse Full Interview*. [Online] Available at: https://www.youtube.com/watch?v=OVs-SlJnzs4

Ray Peat, Clips, 2016b. *Ray Peat on diagnosing hypothyroidism, TSH lab values, circulatory system..* [Online] Available at: https://www.youtube.com/watch?v=ECTtUMvYrEk [Accessed 21 August 2023].

Rupa Health, 2023. *TSH Reference Ranges*. [Online] Available at: https://www.rupahealth.com/lab-tests/vibrant-america-tsh#:~:text=TSH%20Reference%20Ranges,optimal%20for%20most%20healthy%20adults.

Society of Endocrinology, 2020. *Thyroid Gland*. [Online] Available at: https://www.yourhormones.info/glands/thyroid-gland/

Stop the thyroid Madness, 2023. *Rt3-ratio*. [Online] Available at: https://stopthethyroidmadness.com/rt3-ratio/

Sundhed.dk, 2023. *Thyroidea hormoner.* [Online]
Available at:
https://www.sundhed.dk/sundhedsfaglig/lae gehaandbogen/undersoegelser-og-proever/klinisk-biokemi/blodproever/thyroideahormoner/

Vander, A. J., Sherman, J. H. & Luciano, D. S., 2001. *Human Physiology: The Mechanisms of Body Function.* s.l.:McGraw-Hill.

Very Well Health , 2023b. *Antibodies That Contribute to Thyroid Disease.* [Online]
Available at:
https://www.verywellhealth.com/thyroid-antibodies-3231533

Very Well Health, 2023a. *Reading Your Thyroid Blood Test Results.* [Online]
Available at:
https://www.verywellhealth.com/interpret-your-thyroid-test-results-3231840

Wearables, 2022. *Wearables and temperature tracking – the whole story.* [Online]
Available at:
https://www.wareable.com/wearable-tech/wearables-and-temperature-tracking-8878

Wentz, D. I., 2023a. *How To Get Accurate Lab Tests When Taking Thyroid Medications.* [Online] Available at: https://thyroidpharmacist.com/articles/how-to-get-accurate-lab-tests-when-taking-thyroid-medications/

Wentz, D. I., 2023b. Top 10 Thyroid Tests and How to Interpret Them. [Online] Available at: https://thyroidpharmacist.com/articles/top-10-thyroid-tests/

Wilson, D., 2015. Low Body Temperature as an Indicator for Poor Expression of Thyroid Hormone. Integrative Medicine, June, 14(3), p. 24–28.

Benedicte Mai Lerche MSc PhD

Benedicte Mai Lerche MSc PhD

Visit

BiochemNordic.com

Printed in Great Britain
by Amazon